THE SONG PLAY BOOK: SINGING GAMES FOR CHILDREN

Published @ 2017 Trieste Publishing Pty Ltd

ISBN 9780649334858

The Song Play Book: Singing Games for Children by Mary A. Wollaston & C. Ward Crampton

Edited by Trieste Publishing Pty Ltd.
Cover @ 2017

www.triestepublishing.com

MARY A. WOLLASTON & C. WARD CRAMPTON

THE SONG PLAY BOOK: SINGING GAMES FOR CHILDREN

Trieste

THE
SONG PLAY BOOK

SINGING GAMES FOR CHILDREN

COMPILED BY
MARY A. WOLLASTON

EDITED BY
C. WARD CRAMPTON, M.D.
DIRECTOR OF PHYSICAL TRAINING
NEW YORK PUBLIC SCHOOLS

NEW YORK
A. S. BARNES AND COMPANY
1922

PREFACE

These fifty song-plays have been chosen from a great number because of their adaptability to class-room and playground conditions; they also afford a large amount of vigorous exercise in proportion to the small amount of singing demanded. "London Bridge" and games of similar type, though favorites with the children, have been purposely omitted since they are games in which the amount of singing and exercise is not proportionate.

These plays have been used and tested for several years in the New York Training School for Teachers, and have been revised to suit school needs. In several of them a change from the original has been made by introducing a "chorus" between verses so that a vigorous exercise may alternate with a movement more quiet. In a few a slight change in the music has been made where the song covered too great a range for children's voices. The main object has been to make them singable and practical, and where several versions of the same song-play were found, the one chosen was that which seemed most singable and most capable of a smooth dramatization.

An additional index has been arranged in the order of difficulty, the plays being especially suitable for use in grades 1A to 3B inclusive, though they are greatly enjoyed in higher grades and may be used with very good results.

MARY A. WOLLASTON

New York Training School for Teachers.
April, 1917.

INTRODUCTION

The purpose of this collection is to give teachers of little children the means of teaching these delightful forms of physical training so that the best and most happy results may be obtained.

Singing games are the most natural expression of happy childhood. They have been sung, danced and played by countless generations of children, who have handed them down, a priceless heritage.

To the teacher of physical training these games mean a process by which sound and sturdy bodies are made, senses trained, rhythmic expression taught, and fundamental social qualities developed. To the child, however, they mean a happy period of enjoyment. This the teacher should always remember, but should never allow the larger purposes to interfere with a full and intimate participation in the spirit of the occasion.

The present collection is the result of Miss Wollaston's years of careful research and painstaking trial, thoroughly established upon sound pedagogical and hygienic principles.

One of the most valuable features of this work is Miss Wollaston's unique and definite form of presentation, which, while preserving intact the natural tone of the invaluable traditional spirit, yet brings to bear the latest and best in education.

Acknowledgement is gratefully made to Miss Josephine Beiderhase, Assistant Director of Physical Training, for her great help in the preparation of this volume.

C. WARD CRAMPTON,

Director Department of Physical Training,
New York City Public Schools.

ALPHABETICAL INDEX

SONG PLAYS

(*Arranged in Order of Difficulty.*)

DETAILS COMMON TO MANY SONG PLAYS

Types of Formation:

1. *a.* Single circle, all facing centre.
   b. " " one within the ring.
   c. " " several within the ring.
   d. " " one outside the ring.
   e. " " several outside the ring.
   f. " " one inside and one outside the ring.

2. *a.* Single circle, all facing left.
   b. " " one within the ring.
   c. " " several within the ring.

3. Single circle, partners facing each other.

4. *a.* Double circle, all facing centre.
   b. " " all facing left.
   c. " " all facing left, one within the ring.
   d. " " partners facing each other.
   e. " " partners standing side by side and facing in opposite directions.

5. Ranks of three.

6. *a.* Square, one on each side, facing centre.
   b. " two on each side, facing centre.
   c. " one on each corner, all facing centre.
   d. " one couple behind the other, all facing the same direction.

7. A small ring within a large ring, all facing centre.

8. A single line, all standing side by side, facing the same way.

9. *a.* Two parallel lines, facing each other.
   b. Two double parallel lines, facing each other.

Partners: When boys and girls dance together in straight lines, the boy stands on the left of the girl. In circle formation the boy stands on the outside of the circle.

Movement: In song plays of single or double circle formation the movement is at first to the left. Later the direction may be changed.

Steps: The step should be varied when the chorus is repeated. Walking, running, hopping, sliding, and skipping may be used. The rhythm must be quickened for a running step and retarded for the sliding step.

Bow and Curtsey: Boys bow from the hips with arms at sides. In some of the song-plays girls make the "peasant" curtsey, that is, placing right toe close behind the left heel, and bending both knees slightly. In other plays the "minuet" curtsey is indicated. In this one foot is placed well behind the other, the weight is carried on the rear foot, and that knee bent. The skirt is caught with the finger tips and held out at the sides.

THE GALLANT SHIP

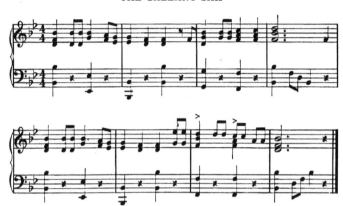

Three times around went the gallant ship,
　And three times around went she;
And three times around went the gallant ship,
　And she sank to the bottom of the sea.

Formation: Single circle, all facing centre with hands joined.

Lines 1, 2 and 3. Sliding step, sideways, left.

Line 4. Players stop and jump very deliberately in place three times. Jump on the words "sank," "bottom," and "sea." On the last jump all sink to the "sitting-on-heels" position.

Repeat from beginning.

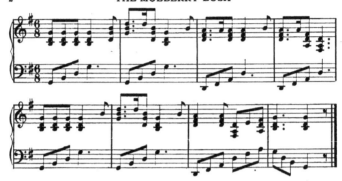

(Introduction and Chorus after each verse.)

Here we go 'round the mulberry bush,
The mulberry bush, the mulberry bush;
Here we go 'round the mulberry bush,
So early in the morning.

VERSES.

1. This is the way we wash our clothes,
We wash our clothes, we wash our clothes,
This is the way we wash our clothes,
So early MONDAY morning.

2. This is the way we iron our clothes, etc.,
So early TUESDAY morning.

3. This is the way we mend our clothes, etc.,
So early WEDNESDAY morning.

4. This is the way we sweep the house, etc.,
So early THURSDAY morning.

5. This is the way we scrub the floor, etc.,
So early FRIDAY morning.

6. This is the way we mix our bread, etc.,
So early SATURDAY morning.

7. This is the way we go to church, etc.,
So early SUNDAY morning.

Formation: Single circle, all facing left with hands joined.

INTRODUCTION AND CHORUS.

Lines 1, 2 and 3. Players dance around the circle to the left with skipping, walking, or sliding steps.

Line 4. Drop hands and turn around to the left in place. Finish facing the centre.

VERSES.

In each verse the action is suggested by the words. The children should make large movements, and be encouraged to move about when sweeping or scrubbing. They return to circle formation during the last line.

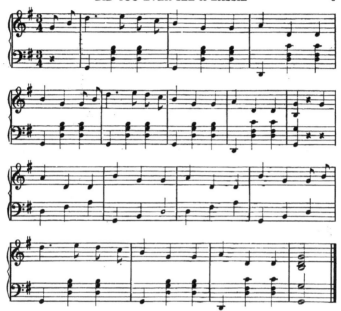

Did you ever see a lassie, a lassie, a lassie,
Did you ever see a lassie do *this* way and *that?*
Do *this* way and *that* way, and *this* way and *that* way,
Did you ever see a lassie do *this* way and *that?*

Formation: Single circle, all facing left with hands joined. A leader stands within the ring.

Lines 1 and 2. Players walk forward around the circle. At the words "do this way and that," the one within the ring demonstrates some movement which the others are to imitate.

Lines 3 and 4. Players stand in place facing centre and perform with the one in the centre the movement shown.

The leader chooses another child to succeed him in the ring and joins the circle.

Suggestions: Activities of the household, of the farm, gymnastic exercises, dance steps, imitations of animals, street games, athletics and industrial activities.

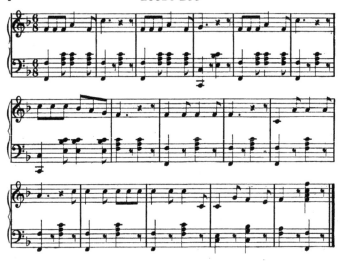

(Introduction and Chorus after each verse.)

Here we dance looby loo,
Here we dance looby light,
Here we dance looby loo,
All on a Saturday night,

1. Put your right hand in,
Put your right hand out,
Give your right hand a shake, shake, shake,
And turn yourself about.

2. Put your left hand in, etc.

3. Put your right foot in, etc.

4. Put your left foot in, etc.

5. Put your head 'way in, etc.

6. Put your whole self in, etc.

Formation: Single circle, all facing left with hands joined.

INTRODUCTION AND CHORUS.

Players dance around the circle to the left with skipping, sliding, walking or running steps.

VERSES.

Players stand facing the centre. The action suggested by the words of the song is given in pantomime. The children should be encouraged to make large and vigorous movements.

For line 3 the movement is made only. three times, that is, on the words, "shake, shake, shake."

In verse 6 the players jump with both feet together into the circle, then out, and three times in place in the same manner.

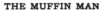

THE MUFFIN MAN

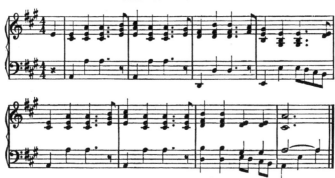

O do you know the muffin man, the muffin man, the muffin man?
O do you know the muffin man who lives in Drury Lane?

O yes, I know the muffin man, the muffin man, the muffin man,
O yes, I know the muffin man who lives in Drury Lane.

Formation: Single circle, facing centre. One child (or more) stands within the ring.

Lines 1 and 2. Players stand in place; the one within the ring stands in front of some one in the circle.

Lines 3 and 4. These two join crossed hands and skip to the right within the ring. Those in the circle face left, join hands and skip around the circle. The two within the ring separate, and each chooses a new partner for a repetition of the game. They then sing "Four of us know the muffin man," later "Eight of us," etc., and finally "All of us know the muffin man."

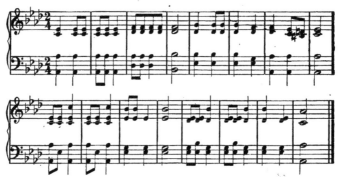

1. Five little chickadees,
   Peeping at the door;
   One flew away,
   And then there were four.

Chorus: Chickadee, chickadee,
           Happy and gay;
           Chickadee, chickadee,
           Fly away.

2. Four little chickadees,
   Sitting on a tree;
   One flew away
   And then there were three.

3. Three little chickadees,
   Looking at you;
   One flew away,
   And then there were two.

4. Two little chickadees,
   Sitting in the sun;
   One flew away,
   And then there was one.

5. One little chickadee,
   Left all alone;
   It flew away,
   And then there were none.

Formation: Single circle, facing centre. Five players crouch in a little group within the circle as "chickadees."

VERSES.

Lines 1 and 2. Children of the circle stand in place and sing.

Lines 3 and 4. A child of the centre group "flies" out to join the circle, and act as leader for the other players during the chorus. He may join the circle any-where and face right or left. The others are obliged to face the same way. In each succeeding verse this is repeated. In this way the centre group is decreased and the circle increased by one each time.

CHORUS.

The players follow the leader around the circle with short, light running steps and a flying movement of the arms.

When the chorus is sung the last time, the players may leave the circle formation and follow the leader as a "flock" of birds.

GARDEN GAME

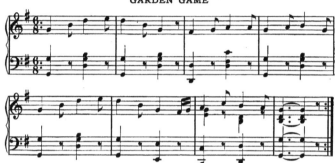

1. This is how we spade the ground,
 In our garden, in our garden,
 This is how we spade the ground,
 In our pretty garden bed.

Chorus: Tra, la, la, la, la, la, la, etc.

2. This is how we rake the ground, etc.

3. This is how we sow the seed, etc.

4. This is how we pull the weeds, etc.

5. This is how we plant the beans, etc.

6. This is how we pick the fruit, etc.

Formation: Single circle, facing centre. A child stands within the ring to lead in the activity.

VERSES.

Players imitate the leader as all sing and dramatize the words.

CHORUS.

Players join hands and skip, walk, run or slide to the left.
Another child is chosen to lead the movement for each verse.

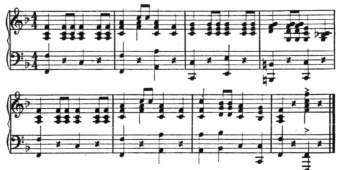

1. One little, two little, three little Indians,
   Four little, five little, six little Indians,
   Seven little, eight little, nine little Indians,
   Ten little Indian boys. (girls)

Chorus: Tra, la, la, la, la, la, etc.

2. Ten little, nine little, eight little Indians,
   Seven little, six little, five little Indians,
   Four little, three little, two little Indians,
   One little Indian boy. (girl)

Formation: Single circle, facing centre. One player stands outside the ring.

FIRST VERSE.

The child outside the circle runs around, touches and numbers ten players, who immediately step into the ring and join hands in a small circle.

CHORUS.

Players in the outer circle join hands and slide to the left. Those in the inner circle slide in the opposite direction.

SECOND VERSE.

Those in the centre return to the outer circle in reverse order on the words "ten, nine, eight," etc.

CHORUS (repeated).

All join hands in a single circle and slide to the left.

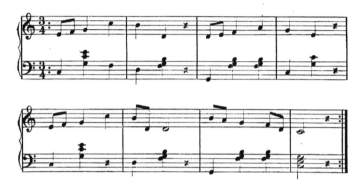

How d'ye do, my partner,
How d'ye do to-day,
Will you dance in the circle?
I will show you the way.

Chorus: Tra, la, la, la, la, la, etc.

Formation: Double circle, partners facing each other.

VERSE.

Line 1. Children in the outside circle make a low curtsey to partners.

Line 2. Children in the inside circle return the curtsey.

Lines 3 and 4. Partners join crossed hands and turn in order to skip side by side.

CHORUS.

Couples skip in a circle.

At the close, children in the outside ring step forward and face a new partner, and the game is repeated.

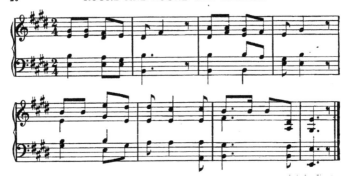

1. Round and round the village,
   Round and round the village,
   Round and round the village,
   As fast as we can go.

2. In and out the windows, etc.,
   As we have done before.

3. Stand and face your partner, etc.,
   And bow before you go.

4. Follow me to London, etc.,
   As we have done before.

Formation: Single circle, facing centre. Several players remain outside the circle.

FIRST VERSE.

The outside players run around the ring to the left.

SECOND VERSE.

Players in the circle join hands and raise arms to form arches, under which the runners pass.

THIRD VERSE.

Each runner steps in front of some one in the circle and bows (4th line). This playmate bows in return. Players in the circle lower arms.

FOURTH VERSE.

The runners and their partners join crossed hands and skip around to the left outside the circle. Players in the circle also skip to the left.

The game is repeated with runners and partners running in line outside the circle. It continues until all have been chosen.

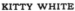

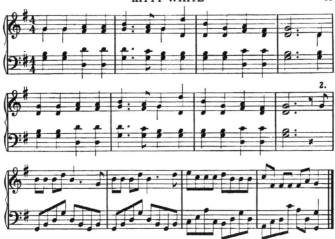

1. Kitty White so slyly comes
   To catch the mousie gray;
   But mousie hears her softly creep,
   And quickly runs away.

2. Run, run, run little mouse,
   Run all around the house;
   For Kitty White is coming near
   And she will catch the mouse, I fear.

Formation: Single circle, facing centre. One player stands within the ring as the mouse; another plays "Kitty White" and moves about outside the ring.

FIRST VERSE.

The players in the circle join hands and walk, slide, skip or run around. Meanwhile, Kitty White is creeping around outside the ring and peeping in at the mouse who moves as the cat advances.

SECOND VERSE.

Those in the circle stand still and clap hands while the mouse runs in and out between players, chased by Kitty White. When the mouse is caught the game is repeated with two new players.

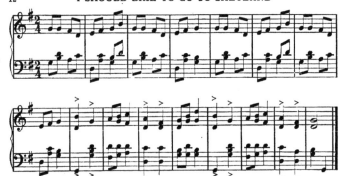

I should like to go to Shetland,
Come and take a ride with me;
I should like to ride a pony,
I can do it, you shall see.
     Gee up!   Come along,
     Gee up!   Come along,
     Gee up!   Come along,
     Whoa!   Back!   Whoa!

Formation: Single circle, facing centre.   One or more players stand within the ring.

Lines 1 and 2.   Those in the circle stand in places and sing.   The player (A) within the ring walks about looking for a pony.

Line 3.   A chooses a child (B) from the circle to be a pony.

Line 4.   A steps behind B and they join hands, B stretching both hands backward and A grasping B's hands.

Lines 5, 6 and 7.   The children forming the circle face left and take the gallop step forward with the left foot.   A and B take the gallop step within the ring in the opposite direction, A driving B.

Line 8.   Those in the circle stop and face the centre.   A stops the pony and draws it backward into place in the circle.

A then rejoins the circle and the game is repeated by other players.   Four or five may stand within the ring at the start of the game.

The circle should face to the right occasionally and take the gallop step with the right foot forward.

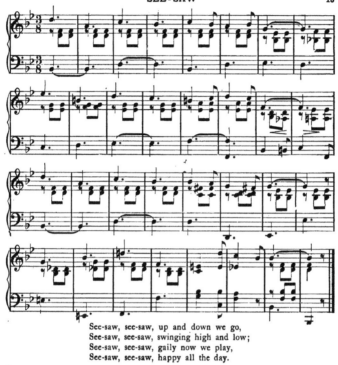

See-saw, see-saw, up and down we go,
See-saw, see-saw, swinging high and low;
See-saw, see-saw, gaily now we play,
See-saw, see-saw, happy all the day.

Formation: Players stand in ranks of three. The ranks may be arranged in a column or in a circle. The middle one of each rank extends the arms sideways and represents the "board." The other two face the centre and with both hands take that of the one in the centre near them.

VERSE.

The one in the centre bends the body alternately left and right while those in the outside lines bend the knees (keeping the body erect). The left line bends first, and then the right.

Players should change places and repeat so all may have each form of exercise.

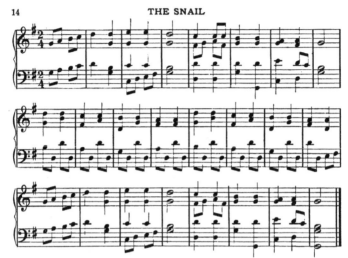

1. Hand in hand you see us well,
   Creep like a snail into his shell.
   Ever nearer, ever nearer,
   Ever closer, ever closer,
   Very snug, indeed, you dwell,
   Snail within your tiny shell.

2. Hand in hand you see us well,
   Creep like a snail out of his shell.
   Ever farther, ever farther,
   Ever wider, ever wider,
   Who'd have thought this little shell
   Could have held us all so well.

Formation: Single circle, all facing left. All except two players join hands; one of these must be the leader.

FIRST VERSE.

The leader winds the class into a spiral formation, ring within ring. He arrives just at the centre as the last line is sung.

SECOND VERSE.

The line unwinds, the leader countermarching through the winding opening of the shell.

Suggestions: Running or skipping may be used when the game is repeated.

A variation for the second verse may be used as follows: The leader draws the line out by going from the centre under the raised arms of the several rings around him, as though passing through a hole in the side of the shell.

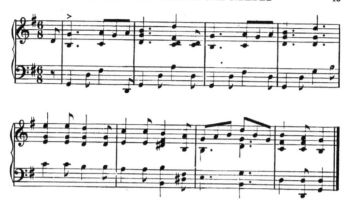

The thread follows the needle,
The thread follows the needle,
In and out the needle goes
As mother mends the children's clothes.

Formation: Single lines of about ten children each. Hands are joined.

Number 10 stands in place. With a light running step number 1 runs down the front of the line and passes under the raised arms of numbers 9 and 10, drawing the children, numbers 1 to 8, after her. After they have passed under the arch numbers 9 and 10, keeping the hands joined, face in the opposite direction and stand with arms crossed on their chests. This starts a kind of "chain stitch." The leader runs to her former position and then passing in front as before, runs between numbers 8 and 9. Number 8 then turns and adds a "stitch" to the chain. This continues and the song is repeated until all the children in line have turned about in this manner. The leader having passed under every arch in the line then turns under her own arm. Result:—all have faced about and all arms are crossed on the chests, making a chain.

At a signal the children all turn about and drop hands quickly, thus unraveling the chain and ripping out the stitches. The game is repeated with a new leader.

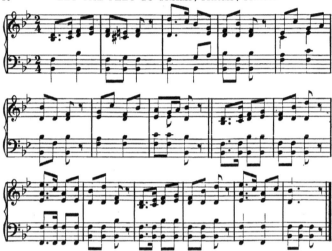

Let the feet go tramp, tramp, tramp,
Let the hands go clap, clap, clap,
Let the finger beckon thee,
Come, dear playmate, skip with me.

Chorus: Tra, la, la, la, la, la, etc.

Formation: Single circle, facing centre. Several children stand within the ring.

VERSE.

Lines 1, 2 and 3. Players suit the action to the words.

Line 4. Those in the centre select partners from the circle and draw them into the ring. They join crossed hands in skaters' fashion.

CHORUS.

Players in the circle join hands and skip to the left. Couples in the centre skip in the opposite direction.

All remain within the ring and select others from the circle during the repetition of the song. The game continues until all in the circle have been chosen.

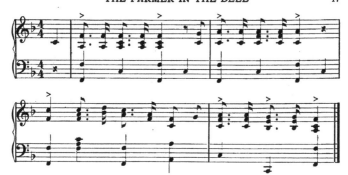

1. The farmer in the dell,
The farmer in the dell,
Heigh-o! the derry-o!
The farmer in the dell.

2. The farmer takes a wife,
The farmer takes a wife,
Heigh-o! the derry-o!
The farmer takes a wife.

3. The wife takes a child, etc.

4. The child takes a nurse, etc.

5. The nurse takes a dog, etc.

6. The dog takes a cat, etc.

7. The cat takes a rat, etc.

8. The rat takes a cheese, etc.

9. The farmer goes away, etc.

10-15. (Wife, child, nurse, dog, cat, rat, all go away in turn.)

16. The cheese stands alone.

Formation: Single circle, all facing centre with hands joined. One child within the ring represents the farmer.

FIRST VERSE.

Players face and skip around to the left. Walking step may be used for alternate verses.

SECOND VERSE.

The farmer selects a child from the circle and draws her into the ring. The circle continues moving to the left.

FOLLOWING VERSES.

The second child in the ring has the privilege of choosing a third child during the third verse. This child will choose a player during the fourth verse, and so on. Those in the centre join hands and move in the opposite direction from the outer circle.

As the game progresses the number within is increased to eight, and after the eighth verse decreased one by one as the words suggest. During the sixteenth verse the child in the centre stands alone. Then the players in the circle stand, and clap hands in rhythm.

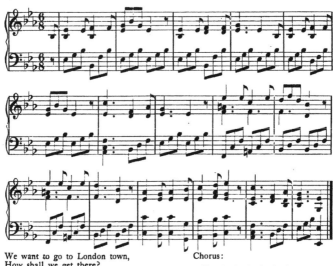

We want to go to London town,
How shall we get there?
We'll go the way the duck goes;
We'll never get there.
   (We'll surely get there).

Chorus:

Tra, la, la, la, la, la, la, etc.
We'll never get there.
   (We'll surely get there).

Formation: Single circle, all facing centre. One player stands within the ring.

VERSE.

Lines 1 and 2. Players stand in place.

Line 3. Centre player sings alone, at the same time imitating a duck walking, by extending arms backward and placing palms together.

Line 4. Those in the circle face left and prepare to "go the way the duck goes."

CHORUS.

Lines 1, 2 and 3. All move around the circle to the left, imitating a waddling duck. The centre player moves also around to the left.

Line 4. All face the centre and stand in place, shaking heads sorrowfully as they sing.

   The game is then repeated with another child in the ring. Substitute for the "duck" a frog, pony, fairy, fish, boat, etc. The last time imitate something that does "get there," as steamship, aeroplane, etc., and sing as indicated above.

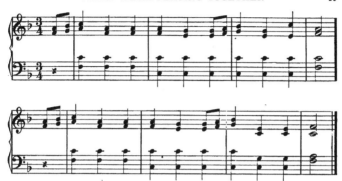

1. When we're playing together
    We are happy and glad,
    In bright or dull weather
    We never are sad.

2. Now tell, little playmate,
    Who has gone from the ring;
    And if you guess rightly,
    We will clap as we sing.

3. Tra, la, la, la, la, etc.

Formation: Single circle, all facing centre with hands joined. One child stands in
    the centre of the ring with closed eyes.

FIRST VERSE.

Players face and skip around to the left. The teacher sends one child from the room
to hide. ·

SECOND VERSE.

Players in the circle stop and face the centre, giving the child in the centre time to
look around and discover who has left the ring. At the end, if the right name is
given, the child in hiding is recalled.

THIRD VERSE.

These two join hands in skaters' fashion and skip within the ring. The others
stand in place, clap hands and sing.

If the name of the child who left the ring cannot be given, this verse is omitted.
The child in hiding is recalled and joins the circle. The child in the centre also re-
turns to the circle.

Another child is sent into the ring and the game is repeated.

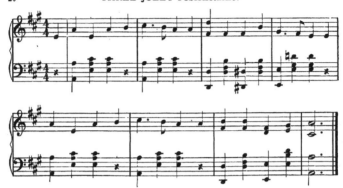

1. There come three jolly fishermen,
   There come three jolly fishermen,
   There come three jolly fishermen,
   Who've just come from the sea.

2. They cast their nets into the sea,
   They cast their nets into the sea,
   They cast their nets into the sea,
   And a jolly old fish caught they.

Formation: Single circle, all facing centre with hands joined. Three players stand in the centre with hands joined, forming a small ring.

FIRST VERSE.

The outer circle skips around to the left; the inner circle to the right.

SECOND VERSE.

Lines 1, 2 and 3. Both circles reverse direction and continue skipping.

Line 4. Each player in the inner circle draws one from the outer circle into the ring. These six join hands.

In this formation the verses are repeated. The first three join the outer circle. The other three remain in the centre for a repetition of the game.

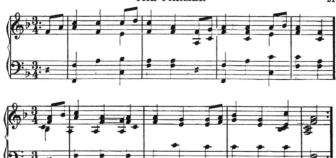

1. Can you tell us how the farmer,
   Can you tell us how the farmer,
   Can you tell us how the farmer,
   Sows grain in his field?

Chorus: O yes, so, so, sows the farmer,
   O yes, so, so, sows the farmer,
   O yes, so, so, sows the farmer,
   Sows grain in his field.

2. Can you tell us how the farmer, etc.,
   Reaps grain in his field?

Chorus:

   O yes, so, so, reaps the farmer, etc.,
   Reaps grain in his field.

3. Can you tell us how the farmer, etc.,
   Stores grain in his barn?

Chorus:

   O yes, so, so, drives the farmer, etc.,
   With grain to his barn.

4. Can you tell us how the farmer, etc.,
   Is threshing his grain?

Chorus:

   O yes, so, so, does the farmer, etc.,
   Thresh grain in his barn.

5. Can you tell us how the farmer, etc.,
   Is grinding his grain?

Chorus:

   O yes, so, so, grinds the farmer, etc.,
   Grinds grain in his mill.

Formation: Single circle, all facing left with hands joined.

VERSES.

Lines 1, 2 and 3. Players skip around the circle.

Line 4. Stop and face the centre.

CHORUS.

Players dramatize the words with large, strong movements as follows: First verse, sowing seed; second verse, cutting with a scythe; third verse, driving a horse (children play in couples, one "driving" the other by means of joined hands); fourth verse, using a flail; fifth verse, turning the handle of a grinder.

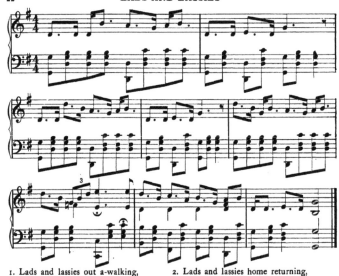

1. Lads and lassies out a-walking,
   Chanced one day to meet;
   First they bowed, then clasping hands,
   Danced with nimble feet.

Chorus: Tra, la, la, la, la, la, etc.

Formation: Single circle, facing centre.

2. Lads and lassies home returning,
   Gaily waved good-bye,   •
   Hoping soon to meet again
   Coming through the rye.

Chorus: Tra, la, la, la, la, la, etc.

Several players stand within the ring.

FIRST VERSE.

Lines 1 and 2. Players in the circle stand and sing; those within the ring walk about looking for a partner.

Lines 3 and 4. Each player within the ring selects a partner from the circle; both bow and join crossed hands.

CHORUS.

Those in the circle join hands and skip around to the left. Couples within the ring skip in the opposite direction.

SECOND VERSE.

Players in the circle stand facing centre as at first. Partners within the ring separate and wave "good-bye." The first players return to the circle; their partners remain in the centre for a repetition of the game.

The game is repeated until all have danced *within* the ring.

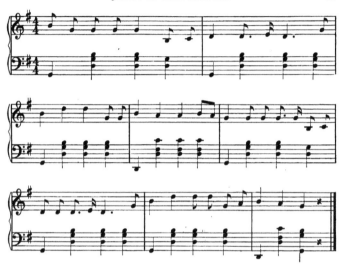

Jolly is the miller who lives by the mill,
The wheel goes round with a right good will;
One hand in the hopper and the other in the sack,
The right steps forward and the left steps back.

Formation: Double circle, all facing left. Partners join inside hands. One player stands in the centre representing the "miller."

Lines 1, 2 and 3. Players march around the circle with a brisk step.

Line 4. A change of partners is made as indicated by the words. The word "back" is the signal for the change. New partners join hands quickly. During the change the "miller" tries to secure a partner by grasping his hand. If he is successful the one left without a partner becomes the "miller," and the game is repeated.

During the progress of the game it is well to stop and change the positions of the players from left to right so that they will have a change of movement forward or backward.

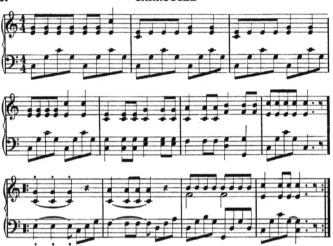

Little children, sweet and gay,
Carrousel is running,
It will run till evening;
Little ones a nickel,
Big ones a dime,
Hurry up, get a mate
Or you'll surely be too late.

   Chorus:

Ha, ha, ha, happy are we,
Anderson and Peterson and Henderson and me!
Ha, ha, ha, happy are we,
Anderson and Peterson and Henderson and me!

Formation: Double circle, all facing centre. Players in the inner circle join hands; those in the outer circle place hands on the shoulders of the one in front.

VERSE.

Lines 1 to 5. Circles move to the left with a slow "follow-step" sideward (step-close).

Lines 6 and 7. The step is shortened and the time quickened.

CHORUS.

Lines 1 and 2. The time is doubled. Players continue moving sideward, now using a sliding follow-step on toes.

Lines 3 and 4. Change direction, that is, sliding step, right.

Players in the two circles exchange places and repeat from the beginning.

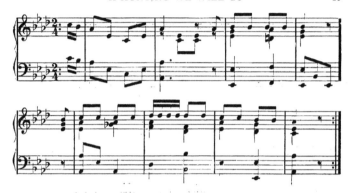

O, a-hunting we will go,
A-hunting we will go,
We'll catch a fox and put him in a box,
And then we'll let him go.

Chorus: Tra, la, la, la, la, la, la, etc.

Formation: Two parallel lines of six players each, facing each other.

VERSE.

Lines 1 and 2. The first (head) couple join crossed hands and skip down between the ranks. The other players stand in place and clap hands in rhythm.

Lines 3 and 4. The couple faces about (turning inward without losing the grasp), and return in the same manner.

CHORUS.

All join crossed hands and skip to the left in a circle, following the leaders. When the head couple reach the place previously occupied by the last couple, they form an arch under which all the others skip.

The second couple now becomes the head. The game is repeated until all have regained their original positions.

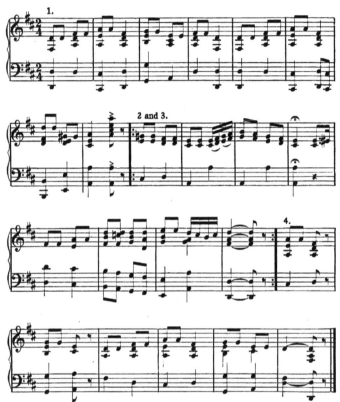

1. Little playmate walk with me,
   On this pleasant sunny day;
   All our little friends we'll see
   Passing on our way.

2. Both your hands now give to me
   And make a pretty bow;
   Playmates all together sing,
   As we go skipping now.

3. Tra, la, la, la, etc.
   (*To the music of the second verse*).

4. Now, good-bye, playmate dear,
   We have had a merry time,
   I will leave you here.

Formation: Players stand in groups or sets of from twelve to sixteen, arranged in two lines facing each other.

FIRST VERSE.

The two head players bow, join inside hands and walk between the lines, bowing and nodding to their friends on both sides until they reach the end of the set.

SECOND VERSE.

Lines 1 and 2. These two join crossed hands and bow.
Lines 3 and 4. They face and prepare to skip between the lines.

THIRD VERSE.

These two skip between the lines and return, while the others clap in rhythm.

FOURTH VERSE.

They separate, bow, and take places at the foot of their respective lines.

The second couple now become the leaders for a repetition of the game. Repeat until all the couples have played.

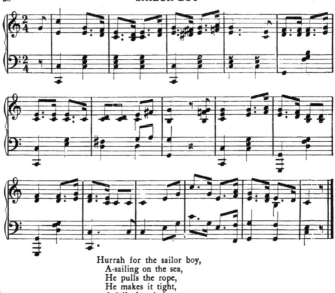

Hurrah for the sailor boy,
A-sailing on the sea,
He pulls the rope,
He makes it tight,
A jolly boy is he.
Hurrah for the sailor boy,
Hurrah for the sailor boy,
Hurrah for the sailor boy,
A-sailing on the sea.

Formation: Single circle, all facing left with hands on hips.

Lines 1 and 2. Players advance with the "step-hop" four times, beginning with the left foot. At the same time place the corresponding hand above the eyes as if "sighting ships."

Lines 3, 4 and 5. Players face centre and make the motion of pulling down a rope three times, using both hands and bending knees.

Lines 6, 7 and 8. On "hurrah" place the left hand on hip and throw the right arm upward and outward. Repeat this with each "hurrah," alternating the movement of the arms.

Line 9. Place hands on hips and turn around to the right in place with three running steps.

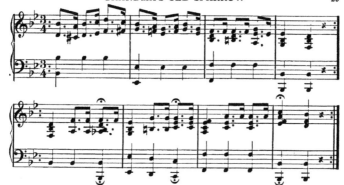

1. Grandma drove her sparrow hitched up to a cart,
   And how to drive she could not tell, O;
   Grandma drove her sparrow hitched up to a cart,
   And how to drive she could not tell, O.

Chorus: This way they stumbled, that way they stumbled,
   Down in the ditch they fell, O;
   This way they stumbled, that way they stumbled,
   Down in the ditch they fell, O.

2. Then the parson started out to drive the sparrow,
   How to drive he could not tell, O;
   Then the parson started out to drive the sparrow,
   How to drive he could not tell, O.

Formation: Single circle, all facing left with hands joined.

VERSES.

   Beginning with the left foot, players run forward, taking three steps to a measure and accenting the first step in each measure.   On the last two words, "tell, O," all face the centre and stamp twice.

CHORUS.

Line 1. . All charge diagonally forward left; recover position; charge diagonally forward right, and recover position.

Line 2.   Bend knees slightly and jump so as to land on the toes with the knees deeply bent at the word "fell."   At the word "O" all come to standing position.

Lines 3 and 4.   Repeat action of lines 1 and 2.

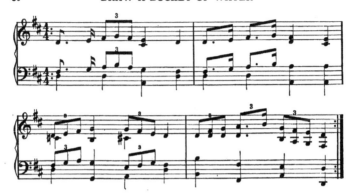

Draw a bucket of water,
For my lady's daughter;
  One in a rush,
  Two in a rush,
Please, little girl, bob under the bush.

Chorus: Tra, la, la, la, la, la, la, etc.

Formation: Players stand in sets of four in the form of a square. Those opposite
    join hands.

VERSE.

Lines 1 to 4. Bracing the feet by placing one foot forward, the couples sway back-
    ward and forward.

Line 5. All raise arms without unclasping hands and place them around one another's
    waists, forming a "bucket."

CHORUS.

In the above position all take eight sliding steps to the left, and then eight to the
right.

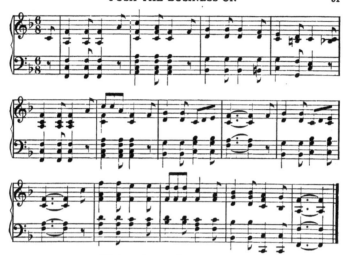

I'll buy a horse and take a gig,
And all the world shall have a jig,
And I'll do all that ever I can
To push the business on,
To push the business on;
And I'll do all that ever I can
To push the business on.

Formation: Single circle, all facing centre with hands joined. Count off in twos for partners.

Lines 1, 2 and 3. Sliding step to the left.

Line 4. All stop and turn around to the left in place, clapping three times.

Line 5. Partners face each other and clap three times.

Lines 6 and 7. Partners place hands on each other's shoulders and turn about in place (starting left) with four skipping steps. Number 1 then passes behind number 2 on his left, with four skipping steps, and takes the next position in the circle.

Hands are joined and the game is repeated from the beginning, number 1 always moving one place to the left.

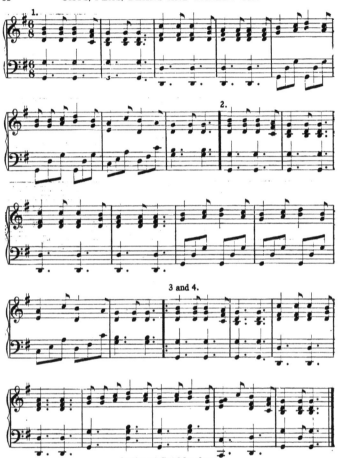

1. Oats, peas, beans and barley grow,
   Oats, peas, beans and barley grow,
   Can you or I or any one know
   How oats, peas, beans and barley grow?

2. Thus the farmer sows his seed;
   Thus he stands and takes his ease;
   Stamps his foot and claps his hands
   And turns around to view his lands.

3. Waiting for a partner,
   Waiting for a partner,
   Open the ring and choose one in,
   While we all gaily dance and sing.

4. Tra, la, la, la, la, la, etc.

Formation: Single circle, all facing left with hands joined. One stands in the centre to impersonate the farmer.

FIRST VERSE.

All walk forward in lively time.

SECOND VERSE.

All stand and dramatize the words.

THIRD VERSE.

All stand and sing while the farmer chooses a partner.

FOURTH VERSE.

Players in the circle skip around to the left; the two within the ring join crossed hands and skip in the opposite direction.

These two remain in the ring and during the third verse in the repetition of the game, each chooses a new partner, etc.

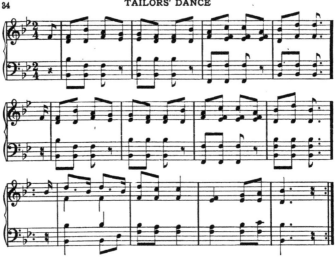

A heart of happiness is mine,
To make a man takes tailors nine;
A heart of happiness is mine,
To make a man takes tailors nine.
With thimble, scissors, needle too,
And thread run through;
With thimble, scissors, needle too,
And thread run through.

Formation: Single circle, all facing left with hands on hips. Count off in twos for
partners.

Lines 1 to 4. Beginning with the left foot, all take eight polka steps (step, close, step)
forward, alternating the feet.

Line 5. Partners face each other; place left hand on hip, bend the right arm with
elbow raised shoulder high in front, and imitate the movement of a pair of
scissors by separating and closing the index and middle fingers. At the same
time touch the left heel sideward and replace. The heel and cutting movements
are done twice.

Line 6. Partners join both hands; extend arms sideways, and take four walking
steps around in place.

Lines 7 and 8. Repeat action of lines 5 and 6, using left hand and right foot.

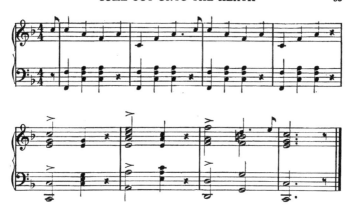

Come out unto the heath to-day,
Come out and join us in our play,
Tra-la, tra-la,
One, two and three.

Formation: Double circle, all facing centre. Those in the inner ring join hands; those in the outer ring place hands on the shoulders of the one in front.

Lines 1 to 3. All take sliding steps to the left. Those in the inner circle take shorter steps than those in the outer circle.

Line 4. At the word "one," those on the outside lift hands and by taking shorter steps catch the shoulders of the player next to their partner as soon as possible.

Repeat taking a new partner in the same way each time. Change direction from time to time, that is, slide right and change left.

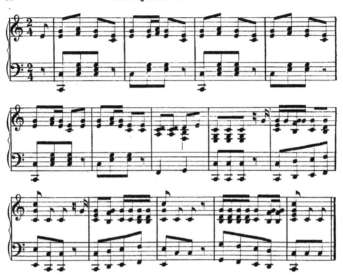

I went into a strange foreign land,
And there I met a queer old man,
And he said to me: "Where goest thee?
And where, young friend, is thy country?"
"I come directly down from curtsey land,
And if you curtsey you can join our band;
Children who are gay come from curtsey land."

Formation: Single circle, all facing centre with hands joined. One player within
the ring impersonates the old man and leads in the action.

Lines 1 to 4. Players slide sideward left. Substitute walking or skipping step.

Lines 5, 6 and 7. Curtsey once during each line as the word is sung.

For other verses, clapping, nodding, stretching, turning, jumping, skipping, skating may be used.

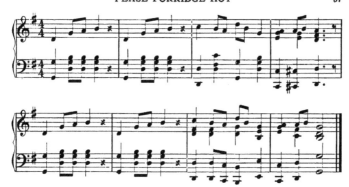

Pease porridge hot, pease porridge cold,
Pease porridge in the pot nine days old;
Some like it hot, some like it cold,
Some like it in the pot nine days' old.

Chorus: Tra, la, la, la, tra, la, la, la, etc.

Formation: Double circle, partners facing.

VERSE.

Line 1. Clap both hands to thighs; clap own hands together; clap partner's hands. Repeat.

Line 2. Clap thighs; clap own hands; clap right hands only; clap own hands; clap left hands only; clap own hands; clap partner's hands.

Line 3 and 4. Repeat action from the beginning. (Counts—1, 2, 3; 1, 2, 3; 1, 2, 3, 4, 5, 6, 7).

CHORUS.

All raise arms sideways (hands joined), and take sixteen sliding steps around the circle to the left; then sixteen in the opposite direction. During the last measure all move to the right and take new partners.

Repeat from the beginning with the new partner.

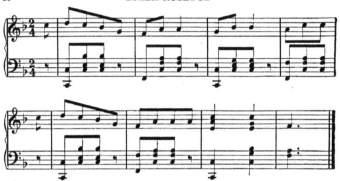

1. Brier Rosebud was a pretty child, pretty child, pretty child;
   Brier Rosebud was a pretty child, a gentle child.

2. She dwelt up in a lonely tower, lonely tower, lonely tower;
   She dwelt up in a lonely tower, a castle tower.

3. One day there came an ugly fay, ugly fay, ugly fay;
   One day there came an ugly fay to that tower.

4. She fell asleep for a hundred years, hundred years, hundred years;
   She fell asleep for a hundred years, as if dead.

5. Great thorny hedges closed her in, closed her in, closed her in;
   Great thorny hedges closed her in, as she slept.

6. But brave Prince Charming cut the thorns, cut the thorns, cut the thorns;
   But brave Prince Charming cut the thorns, one summer morn.

7. Brier Rosebud wakened then from sleep, then from sleep, then from sleep;
   Brier Rosebud wakened then from sleep at the Prince's touch.

8. Brier Rosebud was the Prince's bride, Prince's bride, Prince's bride;
   And merrily they danced away, side by side.

Formation: Two circles, one within the other. All players stand facing centre with hands joined.

The larger, outer circle represents the hedge; the inner one, containing only six or seven players, represents the castle. Within the inner ring a player impersonates the Princess. Two others, a Prince and a Fairy, walk outside the hedge.

FIRST VERSE.

Players in both circles walk around to the left.

SECOND VERSE.

All stand. Players in the inner circle raise arms high, hands joined.

THIRD VERSE.

The ugly Fairy slips into the castle and, waving a wand, casts a spell over the Princess, who falls asleep.

FOURTH VERSE.

The Princess remains asleep. The two circles walk around to the left as at first.

FIFTH VERSE.

All stand. Players in the outer circle raise arms high with fingers pointing, to represent a hedge.

SIXTH VERSE.

The Prince runs around the hedge cutting the thorns by striking lightly the uplifted hands, which drop at his touch. He then enters the castle and touches the Princess, who awakens and rises.

SEVENTH VERSE.

The Prince and Princess join crossed hands ready to dance side by side. Those in the inner circle drop hands and move outward to enlarge the circle.

EIGHTH VERSE.

The Prince and Princess skip within the inner ring, and the circles skip around to the left.

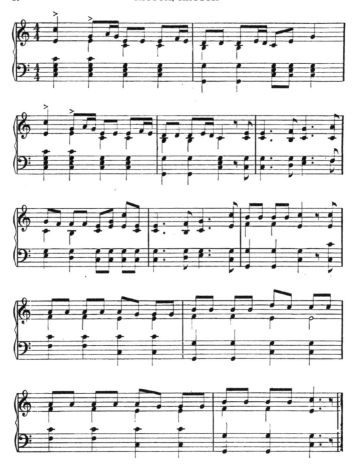

RITSCH, RATSCH (Continued).

Ritsch, ratsch, filebom-bom-bom,
Filebom-bom-bom, filebom-bom-bom;
Ritsch, ratsch, filebom-bom-bom,
Filebom-bom-bom, filebom.
Miss Henderson, Miss Henderson, Miss Henderson,
Miss Henderson, and little Ann Marie;
They washed themselves in ocean water, ocean water, ocean water;
Washed themselves in ocean water, ocean water clear.

Formation: Groups of four. Players stand on the corners of a square, all facing centre. Partners stand on diagonal corners. Hands are on hips. For convenience in teaching, number children 1, 2, 3 and 4.

Line 1. All clap hands twice; then hop on the right foot and place left heel forward.

Line 2. Hop on left foot and place right heel forward; hop on right foot and place left heel forward.

Lines 3 and 4. Repeat action of lines 1 and 2.

Line 5. As "Miss Henderson" is sung the first time, numbers 1 and 2 bow, bending from the hips with the heels together. At the same time their opposites 3 and 4 curtsey (touch right toe behind the left heel and bend both knees). As "Miss Henderson is sung the second and third time in quicker rhythm numbers 1 and and 2 curtsey, and 3 and 4 bow.

Line 6. As "Miss Henderson" is sung, numbers 1 and 2 bow, and 3 and 4 curtsey as at first. At the words "little Ann Marie" clap hands three times.

Lines 7 and 8. All face left. Beginning with the left foot dance seven polka steps forward. Finish facing centre, stamping on the word "clear."

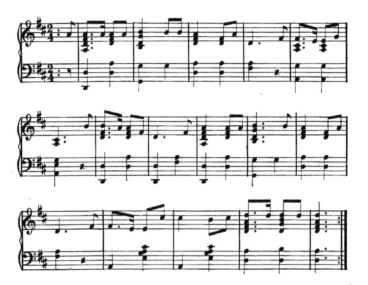

Our little girls, we know,
  When a dancing they go,
Would like a girl to know,
  With whom to dance, just so.
And if you will be a partner to me,
Just put your hand in mine
And dance so merrily.

Chorus: O bom fa ral la, bom fa ral la,
        Bom fa ral la la,
        O bom fa ral la la,
        O bom fa ral la la;
        And if you will be a partner to me,
        Just put your hand in mine
        And dance so merrily.

OUR LITTLE GIRLS (Continued).

Formation: Single circle, all facing left with hands joined. Several players stand within the ring.

VERSE.

Lines 1 to 4. Players walk forward with a brisk step and swinging arms. Those within the ring walk in the opposite direction.

Line 5. Players within the ring choose partners from the circle, which continues moving left.

Lines 6 and 7. Partners within the ring join hands and walk in the opposite direction from the circle, as at first.

CHORUS.

Lines 1 and 2. Players in the circle skip forward; partners within the ring face each other and turn rapidly in place with skipping steps, knees high.

Lines 3 and 4. *All* reverse direction.

Lines 5, 6 and 7. All walk as at first, that is, those in the circle to the left, and those within the ring to the right.

Those chosen remain in the ring; the others return to the circle and the game is repeated.

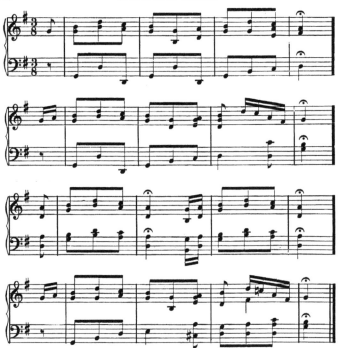

The cuckoo is singing,
The May, it is here;
In the field and the forest,
The green doth appear.
Then dance, children, dance,
While the sky, it is blue;
Turn round and turn under
While I go with you.

SWISS MAY DANCE (Continued).

Formation: Double circle, all facing left with right hands joined. The left hand holds the skirt. This position of the hands is retained throughout the dance.

Step: Raise and point the left toe forward at the beginning of every phrase. Count "and" for this.

Lines 1 and 2. Players start with the left foot and run forward nine steps; put the right foot behind on the tenth count (the word "here"); face partner and make a deep curtsey (minuet).

Lines 3 and 4. Repeat, running in the opposite direction. Curtsey at the word "appear."

Line 5. Partners exchange places with three running steps; face each other and curtsey.

Line 6. Return to place with three steps and curtsey as before.

Line 7. Partners turn each other around in place with six running steps.

Line 8. The one on the outside turns inward and about under her own arm and advances to the next player, who extends her right hand in welcome. These two become partners for a repetition of the game.

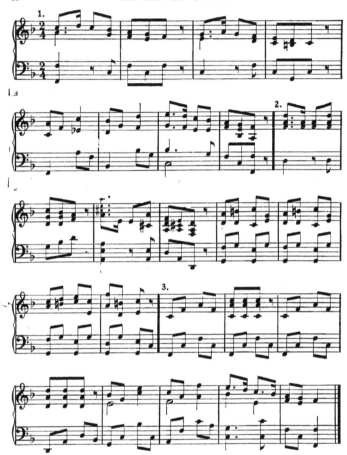

1. Little playmate, dance with me,
   Both your hands now give to me;
   Heel and toe, away we go,
   Up and down the merry row.

2. Tra, la, la, la, la, la, la, etc.

3. With your feet go tap, tap, tap,
   With your hands go clap, clap, clap,
   Heel and toe, away we go,
   Up and down the merry row.

For a repetition of the game, verse 3 is as follows:

3. With your head go nip, nip, nip,
   With your fingers snip, snip, snip,
   Heel and toe, away we go,
   Round and round so merry, oh.

Formation: Players stand in groups or sets of eight or ten, arranged in two lines, facing each other.

FIRST VERSE.

Lines 1 and 2. Head couple make a deep curtsey (minuet), holding skirts out at sides; then join crossed hands and face playmates.

Line 3. Place outside heel forward, then outside toe backward, and take polka step (hop-slide, close, step) with the same foot.

Line 4. Partners turn inward and about, and take heel-and-toe polka once with the inside foot in this direction.

SECOND VERSE.

Head couple raise arms and make an arch; other players skip through the arch, turn to the left and return to places. The head couple follows and remains at the foot.

THIRD VERSE.

Lines 1 and 2. All dramatize the words.

Lines 3 and 4. All face toward the head of the set and dance two heel-and-toe polka steps, as the leaders did in the first verse, beginning with the outside foot.

Repeat from the beginning, using the alternate third verse.

Alternate third verse.

Lines 1 and 2. All dramatize the words.

Lines 3 and 4. Partners join hands and dance heel-and-toe polka, beginning with the left foot and turning partner once around in place.

THE RILL

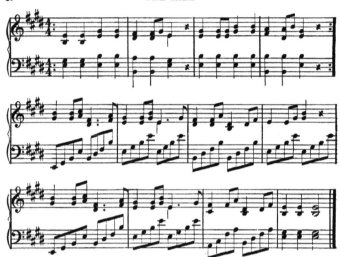

One and two and three, four and five,
Now we again the Rill revive;
One and two and three, four and five,
Now we again the Rill revive.
Dance we now the Rill all right,
And dance we now till it grows light;
Dance we now the Rill all right,
And dance we now from morn till night.

Formation: Players stand in groups of four. In each group one couple (partners)
stands behind the other couple. Partners join inside hands; outside hands are
joined with the outside hands of the other couple, thus forming a square.

Line 1. All take two polka steps (slide, close, step) forward, beginning with the outside foot.

Line 2. All take four jig steps (step-hop), the forward couple breaking inside grasp,
swinging outward and into place behind the rear couple, who move forward
with four jig steps and become the head couple. The couple now in the rear
join inside hands.

Lines 3 to 8. Repeat steps of lines 1 and 2 three times.
Repeat all.

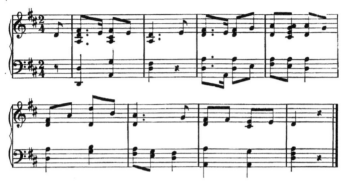

1. To-day's the first of May,
   To-day's the first of May, May, May;
   To-day's the first of May,
   To-day's the first of May.

2. Good-bye, farewell, my friend,
   We'll meet again some day, some day;
   We'll meet again some day,
   Before the first of May.

Formation: Double circle, all facing left. Partners join inside hands and place the outside hand on hip.

First Verse.

All dance eight polka steps forward, beginning with the outside foot and turning toward and from each other alternately. Swing the arms backward and forward vigorously.

Second Verse.

Line 1. Partners face each other and shake right hands. At the word "friend" they slap right hands.

Lines 2 and 3. Outer circle skips forward around the circle; inner circle turns and skips in the opposite direction.

Line 4. Each player stops at the player just in front of his former partner; these two join hands and face forward for a repetition of the game.

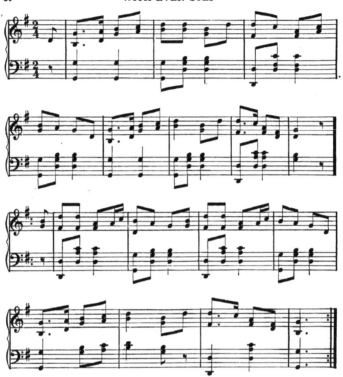

A maid is walking in the ring with even step and merry swing,
She's seeking for a partner to join her in the ring;
Tra-la-la-la-la-la-la-la-la, tra-la-la-la-la-la-la-la-la,
The maid has found a partner to join her in the ring;
Tra-la-la-la-la-la-la-la-la, tra-la-la-la-la-la-la-la-la,
The maid has found a partner to join her in the ring.

WITH EVEN STEP (Continued).

Formation: Single circle, all facing left with hands joined. Several players take places within the ring.

Lines 1 and 2. Players in the circle walk forward in lively time; those within, walk in the opposite direction. At the word "partner" those in the centre draw a partner into the ring.

Line 3. Players in the circle skip around to the left; partners in the centre face each other, and with hands on hips take eight kicking steps, raising left and right foot forward alternately in quick time, keeping the knees straight and the toes pointed downward.

Line 4. Outer circle continues skipping; partners in the centre join hands and skip about in place, turning to the left.

Line 5. Outer circle changes direction; those within the ring repeat eight "kicking" steps.

Line 6. Outer circle continues skipping; partners in the centre join hands and skip to the right.

When the game is repeated, those chosen as partners remain in the ring and the others return to the circle.

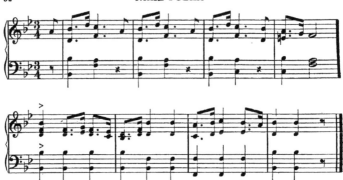

A little while we linger here,
With many a joy and many a fear;
Hey! little Brownies, come and frolic,
Let us always be merry.

Formation: Single circle, all facing centre, with hands on hips. One child stands
in the centre.

Lines 1 and 2. The centre (A) stands in front of a player (B) in the circle, invit-
ing her to dance. On the words "while," "here," "joy" and "fear" all dance the
Bleking step four times, alternating left and right. (Bleking step—hop on the
left foot, bending the left knee, and place the right heel forward).

Lines 3 and 4. At "Hey" all clap hands; A then faces about with hands on hips; B
places hands on A's shoulders and they run twelve steps to another player (C).
At the same time those in the circle take twelve running steps in place.

Lines 1 and 2. Repetition of verse. In this position all dance four Bleking steps.

Lines 3 and 4. A and B both face about on "Hey." Thus B is the leader. A places
hands on B's shoulders; C places hands on A's shoulders, and all three run in
line to another player (D).

The game continues in this manner until all have been chosen from the circle and
have entered the running line. The first runner now grasps the shoulders of the last
girl, thus making a complete circle. Lines 3 and 4 may be repeated several times
while players continue running in circle formation.

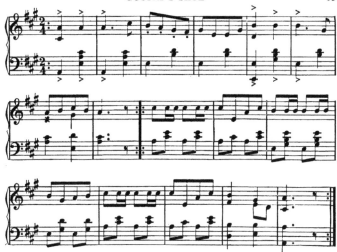

Gustaf's skol! (*Gustavus' toast.*)
There is no better skol than this;
Gustaf's skol!
The best old skol there is.

Chorus: Tra, la, la, la, la, la, etc.

Formation: Players are divided into sets of eight as for a quadrille, that is, four
couples arranged so as to form a square. Partners join inside hands and place
other hand on hip.

VERSE.

Lines 1 and 2. Head couples take three walking steps toward each other, bow, and
take three steps back to place.

Lines 3 and 4. Side couples do the same.

Repeat lines 1 to 4. Action is the same.

CHORUS.

Side couples form an arch. The head couples walk to centre, separate and, taking inside hand of opposite, walk through the arch nearest them. Returning to place
they clap hands once, and with both hands turn partners around in place with three
polka steps. Head couples make arches and the sides pass under in the same manner.

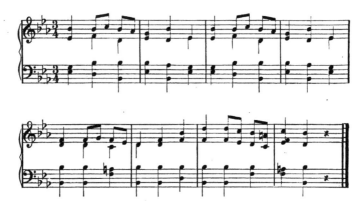

1. Seven jolly girls are in a ring,
   Seven jolly girls are in a ring,
   Jollier girls there can't be seen
   'Mongst all our playmates.

2. Girls, now, oh turn yourselves about,
   Girls, now, oh turn yourselves about;
   Come, choose you each a partner out,
   Tra, la, la, la, la, la, la.

3. Now am I thine, if thou art mine,
   Now am I thine, if thou art mine;
   Take then the hand I give as sign
   That I am now thy partner.

4. Now we are happy all the day,
   Now we are happy all the day;
   So let us sing and dance and play,
   Tra, la, la, la, la, la, la.

Formation: Two circles, one within the other, all facing centre. The inner circle consists of seven players.

FIRST VERSE.

Players in the outer circle walk around to the left in lively rhythm; those in the inner circle walk to the right.

SECOND VERSE.

Outer circle continues walking in the same direction. Players in the inner circle stop, clap hands, face outward, join hands again and move in the opposite direction from the outer circle.

THIRD VERSE.

Players in the inner ring drop hands and choose partners from the outer circle, drawing the chosen one into the ring with both hands.

FOURTH VERSE.

Lines 1 and 2. With hands joined couples turn about in place with four skipping steps, starting with the left foot.

Lines 3 and 4. In the same position take four skipping steps, turning around to the right.

The seven chosen remain in the centre; the first seven join the outer circle and the game is repeated.

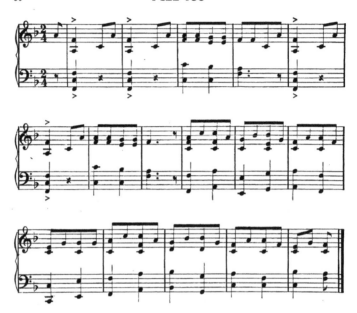

I see you, I see you,

Tra, la, la, la, la, la, la.

I see you, I see you,

Tra, la, la, la, la, la.

You see me and I see you,

And you take me and I take you;

You see me and I see you,

And you take me and I take you.

Formation: Two double ranks facing each other, about five feet apart. Those in the front rank place hands on hips; those in the rear rank place hands on the shoulders of those in front.

Line 1. Those in the front rank stand still; those in the rear rank bend heads first left then right, playing "peek-a-boo" with rear players in the opposite rank.

Line 2. Bend head four times, left and right alternately.

Line 3. Bend head twice only; first left, then right.

Line 4. Bend head twice, alternating as before, then stand erect.

Line 5. All players in the rear ranks clap hands once and, passing to the left, run forward to meet the playmate from the opposite side; these two join hands.

Line 6. Couples now in the centre turn around in place with sliding steps, leaning away from partner.

Line 7. Couples separate with a sharp clap on the first note, and join hands with original partner.

Line 8. Partners slide once around in place, finishing with the position of the ranks reversed, that is, those of the front rank in the rear.

Repeat from the beginning in this formation.

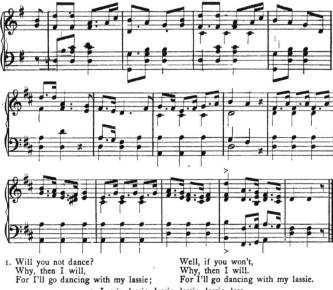

1. Will you not dance?   Well, if you won't,
Why, then I will,   Why, then I will.
For I'll go dancing with my lassie;   For I'll go dancing with my lassie.

2. Lassie, lassie, lassie, lassie, lassie, lass,
Lassie, lassie, lassie, lassie, lassie, lass,
Hey! dance with my lassie.

Formation: Single circle, partners facing each other. Hands are on hips.

FIRST VERSE.

Line 1. Place the right toe forward, execute a half-turn left (180) on both toes; bend the right knee and bow to the neighbor behind, keeping the left toe pointed.

Line 2. Execute a half-turn right and bow to partner, bending left knee and pointing right toe.

Lines 3 to 6. Repeat action of lines 1 and 2, three times.

SECOND VERSE.

Lines 1 and 2. Beginning with the left foot, players take twelve kicking steps (leg raised forward with toes pointed and feet kept near the floor), alternating the feet.

Line 3. At "Hey" clap hands with partner and turn around in place with three quick running steps, stamping as the feet close on the fourth count.

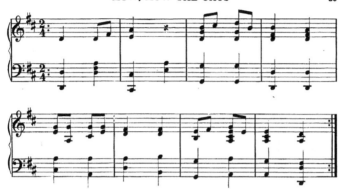

1. Mow, mow the oats,
Who shall do the binding?
I've a merry partner,
But I cannot find him.

Chorus: Tra, la, la, la, etc.

2. Bind, bind the oats,
Who shall do the threshing?
When the harvest work is done
Then I'll surely find him.

Formation: Double circle, consisting of twelve couples. Partners stand side by side, facing in opposite directions.

FIRST VERSE.

All walk forward until partners meet.

CHORUS.

Partners join hands, extend arms sideways, and take eight sliding steps, moving left around the circle; then eight to the right.

SECOND VERSE.

Formation as at first. Players skip forward until they meet again, making a "grand chain" (right and left hands given alternately to dancers encountered in skipping around the circle).

CHORUS.

Action as before.

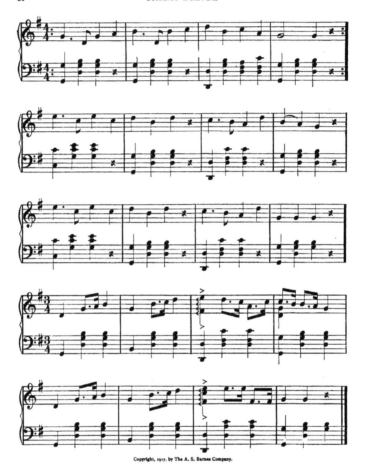

CHAIN DANCE (Continued).

I am wandering here alone,
I'm looking for my partner;
I am wandering here alone,
I'm looking for my partner.
Now at last I find her here,
She who is my partner;
Come, my friend, and dance with me,
Sing and dance around with me.

Chorus: Tra, la, la, la, la, la, la, etc.

Formation: Single circle; partners facing. Join right hands and place left hand on hip.

Lines 1 to 4. All walk forward around the circle, partners advancing in opposite directions in a "grand chain," grasping right and left hands alternately.

Line 5. Retain the right hand grasped just at this time, place left hand on hip. With this girl as a partner, stand and swing clasped hands from side to side in rhythm with the music.

Line 6. Join left hands also, so that players are standing side by side in skaters' fashion.

Line 7. Walk forward four steps, swinging arms up and down with the music.

Line 8. Partners face each other, extend arms sideways, shoulder high, hands joined, and turn around in place with four steps.

CHORUS.

Formation: Double circle, all facing left. Partners join inside hands and place other hand on hip.

Starting with the outside foot dance two polka-steps forward; in waltz position turn about in place with the "step-hop" four times (hop-waltz). Repeat two polka-steps forward and the hop-waltz.

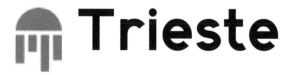

Trieste Publishing has a massive catalogue of classic book titles. Our aim is to provide readers with the highest quality reproductions of fiction and non-fiction literature that has stood the test of time. The many thousands of books in our collection have been sourced from libraries and private collections around the world.

The titles that Trieste Publishing has chosen to be part of the collection have been scanned to simulate the original. Our readers see the books the same way that their first readers did decades or a hundred or more years ago. Books from that period are often spoiled by imperfections that did not exist in the original. Imperfections could be in the form of blurred text, photographs, or missing pages. It is highly unlikely that this would occur with one of our books. Our extensive quality control ensures that the readers of Trieste Publishing's books will be delighted with their purchase. Our staff has thoroughly reviewed every page of all the books in the collection, repairing, or if necessary, rejecting titles that are not of the highest quality. This process ensures that the reader of one of Trieste Publishing's titles receives a volume that faithfully reproduces the original, and to the maximum degree possible, gives them the experience of owning the original work.

We pride ourselves on not only creating a pathway to an extensive reservoir of books of the finest quality, but also providing value to every one of our readers. Generally, Trieste books are purchased singly - on demand, however they may also be purchased in bulk. Readers interested in bulk purchases are invited to contact us directly to enquire about our tailored bulk rates. Email: customerservice@triestepublishing.com

You May Also Like

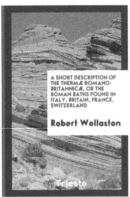

ISBN: 9780649353040
Paperback: 92 pages
Dimensions: 6.14 x 0.19 x 9.21 inches
Language: eng

A short description of the thermæ Romano-Britannicæ, or the Roman baths found in Italy, Britain, France, Switzerland

Robert Wollaston

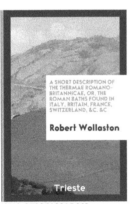

ISBN: 9780649345663
Paperback: 88 pages
Dimensions: 6.14 x 0.18 x 9.21 inches
Language: eng

A Short Description of the Thermae Romano-Britannicae, Or, The Roman Baths found in Italy, Britain, France, Switzerland, &C. &C

Robert Wollaston

www.triestepublishing.com

You May Also Like

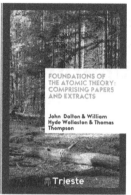

Foundations of the Atomic Theory: Comprising Papers and Extracts

John Dalton & William Hyde Wollaston & Thomas Thompson

ISBN: 9780649279999
Paperback: 60 pages
Dimensions: 6.14 x 0.12 x 9.21 inches
Language: eng

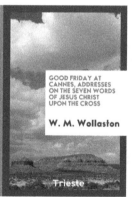

Good Friday at Cannes, addresses on the seven words of Jesus Christ upon the Cross

W. M. Wollaston

ISBN: 9780649350582
Paperback: 91 pages
Dimensions: 6.14 x 0.19 x 9.21 inches
Language: eng

www.triestepublishing.com

You May Also Like

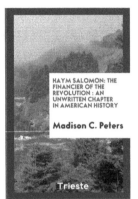

Haym Salomon: The Financier of the Revolution : an Unwritten Chapter in American History

Madison C. Peters

ISBN: 9781760570170
Paperback: 56 pages
Dimensions: 6.14 x 0.12 x 9.21 inches
Language: eng

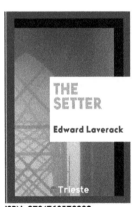

The setter

Edward Laverack

ISBN: 9781760570309
Paperback: 90 pages
Dimensions: 6.14 x 0.19 x 9.21 inches
Language: eng

www.triestepublishing.com

You May Also Like

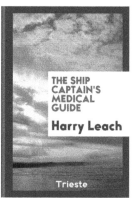

The Ship Captain's Medical Guide

Harry Leach

ISBN: 9781760570620
Paperback: 120 pages
Dimensions: 6.14 x 0.25 x 9.21 inches
Language: eng

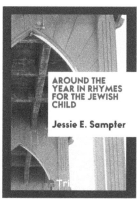

Around the Year in Rhymes for the Jewish Child

Jessie E. Sampter

ISBN: 9781760570712
Paperback: 104 pages
Dimensions: 5.83 x 0.22 x 8.27 inches
Language: eng

Find more of our titles on our website. We have a selection of thousands of titles that will interest you. Please visit

www.triestepublishing.com

Lightning Source UK Ltd.
Milton Keynes UK
UKHW02f0601010618
323575UK00005B/309/P